Alternative Treatments of Post-traumatic Stress Disorder (PTSD)

Safe, effective and affordable approaches and how to use them

James Lake, MD

This book is dedicated to my best friend and soul mate, Nicole Asselborn, MD, with gratitude for invaluable advice on the right scope and 'voice' for this project, and for creating the lovely image on the cover.

Contents

Disclaimer

The information provided in this book is intended to provide helpful information on the treatment of post-traumatic stress disorder (PTSD) and does not constitute medical advice. The publisher and author are not responsible for any specific health needs that may require medical supervision, and are not liable for any damages or negative consequences from any treatment, action or application to any person reading or using the information in this book. References to internet resources are provided for informational purposes only and do not constitute endorsement of any websites or other sources. Readers should be aware that the websites listed in this book may change.

Part I: Introduction

What this book is about

My chief goal in writing this book and the others in the series was to create a practical low-cost resource on safe and effective alternative treatments of mental health problems including herbals, vitamins and other natural supplements, mind-body approaches, and energy therapies.

The subject of this book is post-traumatic stress disorder (PTSD). You will learn about a variety of safe and effective alternative treatments of PTSD. If you are currently struggling with symptoms of PTSD, taking a medication that isn't helping, experiencing side effects, or you can't afford to continue taking a medication that *is working* this book provides valuable information about alternative treatments of PTSD and practical strategies for how to use them.

If you've had PTSD in the past and you are no longer experiencing debilitating symptoms of PTSD, this book will help you create a wellness plan that fits your lifestyle and your budget. By the time you finish reading you'll be able to create an individualized care plan adapted to your needs, preferences and budget. Just as important, you will learn how to *think about* your mental health care in a more holistic way.

How to use this book

This book was *written to give you the maximum amount of information in the least amount of time*. The last section of the book is a summary of the most important points. I've provided links to valuable internet resources to help you find quality brands of natural supplements and other alternative treatments, important safety information and professional help if you think you need it.

If you are a mental health professional this book provides concise, jargon-free summaries of scientifically validated alternative treatments you can use when advising clients about safe, effective treatments of PTSD.

Alternative and integrative medicine defined

Alternative medicine—sometimes called 'complementary and alternative medicine or CAM—consists of approaches that are currently not used in mainstream Western medicine (also called 'biomedicine' and 'allopathic medicine'). Examples of CAM include acupuncture, herbs and other natural supplements, so-called 'energy' therapies such as Healing Touch, and others.

Integrative medicine is a rapidly growing model of care that takes a middle ground between Western medicine as conventionally practiced and CAM. Integrative medicine:

- is a person-centered approach

- that takes account of the needs and preferences of each unique person

- that focuses on maintaining optimal health and treating symptoms

- uses both conventional mainstream approaches like medications and psychotherapy, and complementary and alternative (CAM) therapies like herbal medicines and acupuncture

- is based on the *best available* scientific evidence

Integrative mental health care defined

Integrative mental health care is a specialized area of integrative medicine aimed at helping each person find safe, appropriate and effective treatments for their mental health problem taking into account their unique symptoms, values, preferences and circumstances.

Integrative mental health care often includes advice on life-style changes that require on-going commitment to improving health and mental health such as changing your diet, exercising more, sleeping better, and using relaxation techniques to reduce stress. In addition to lifestyle changes integrative mental health care may include advice on select herbals, vitamins and other natural supplements when there is evidence for both their safety and effectiveness. Finally, Integrative mental health care may include prescription medications or other conventionally used treatments.

If this is the first time you've heard about integrative mental health care and want to find out more before trying a new treatment for anxiety, I encourage you to download the first book in the series to learn more. This book is available as a free download and will give you an overview of essential concepts and methods in integrative mental health care.

About Dr. Lake's background and qualifications

I completed my medical training at University of California, Irvine, and did my residency in adult psychiatry at Stanford University Hospital. I am board-certified by the American Board of Psychiatry and Neurology, and I have practiced psychiatry for more than 20 years in diverse settings. I've had extensive experience taking care of patients in hospitals, clinics, emergency rooms and in my private practice. I have been a student of herbal medicine for decades and I am certified in medical acupuncture and in EEG biofeedback. I previously served on the teaching faculty at Stanford University Hospital and I am currently an adjunct clinical assistant professor in the Department of Psychiatry at University of Arizona College of Medicine. I've taught physicians and other mental health professionals about integrative mental healthcare at national and international conferences. I publish a column on integrative mental health care in *Psychiatric Times,* a leading trade publication for mental health professionals and I am a frequent blogger on Psychology Today. I've authored numerous articles and chapters in medical journals and textbooks, and I've written, co-authored or edited five textbooks covering the philosophy, theory and practice of integrative mental healthcare.

I've been involved in national and international efforts to establish integrative mental healthcare as a new medical sub-specialty in its own right. I founded and previously chaired an initiative aimed at changing mental health care into a more effective, safer and more person-centered model of care: the American Psychiatric Association Caucus on Complementary and Integrative Medicine. An important goal of the Caucus is the development of expert resources for educating and training psychiatrists in the safe, *evidence-based* uses of non-medication treatments for treating PTSD, anxiety, depression and the other mental health problems covered in the book series.

What to do if you have severe symptoms of PTSD

Severe symptoms of PTSD include:

- Repetitive intrusive memories of a traumatic experience (flashbacks)

- Heightened autonomic arousal (e.g. perspiration, rapid breathing, elevated heart rate)

- Psychic 'numbing' (a general feeling of mental and emotional 'dullness')

- Frequent nightmares about a traumatic experience

- Hyper-vigilance (an exaggerated sense of constantly being 'on guard' for danger)

- Dissociative symptoms (difficulty knowing whether your body or the environment is 'real')

- Auditory or visual hallucinations

If you are having frequent flashbacks, nightmares, dissociative symptoms or other PTSD symptoms that are interfering with your ability to function day to day, I encourage you to consult with a psychiatrist or other mental health provider as soon as possible.

When your situation has improved the treatments described in this book may help you feel and function better. If you are experiencing severe symptoms of PTSD or have another serious mental health problem you may need to take a medication in order to function in the workplace, at home or in a relationship.

Part II: Understanding and treating PTSD from a holistic point of view

Understanding PTSD

The information in the following sections will help you understand your PTSD symptoms better and give you the tools you need to develop a safe, effective and affordable treatment plan. You will learn about typical symptoms of PTSD as well as medical and mental health problems that sometimes occur together with this condition.

PTSD is a severe anxiety disorder that occurs following *direct* or *indirect* exposure to trauma. In cases of *direct* exposure to trauma symptoms of PTSD develop after a potentially life-threatening situation such as a serious injury, physical assault or *threat* of assault, torture or rape. PTSD may also result from *indirect exposure* to trauma such as witnessing events that threaten the lives of others but do not directly affect the observer, or learning about a life-threatening event, especially one that affected a family member or friend.

Symptoms of PTSD may begin within days following exposure to trauma or onset may be delayed months or years. Approximately one half of individuals diagnosed with PTSD recover fully within 3 months without treatment however many individuals experience a more prolonged course of illness that may severely impair functioning and become a chronic debilitating condition. Factors associated with increased risk of more severe or prolonged forms of PTSD include previous exposure to trauma, history of mental illness prior to trauma, lower socioeconomic class or less education, younger age, female gender, the severity of the trauma, and the presence of dissociative symptoms during the traumatic experience. Traumatized individuals may be severely impaired by their symptoms and unable to function at work, in school, in relationships or in other social contexts.

Symptoms of *psychic numbing* typically start immediately following exposure to trauma. Other symptoms usually emerge in the days and weeks following trauma including repetitive intrusive memories of the traumatic experience (flashbacks), autonomic arousal (perspiration, rapid breathing, and elevated heart rate), recurring nightmares, and hyper-vigilance. Traumatized individuals actively avoid situations that remind them of the traumatic event, may have amnesia of the traumatic event, and often experience profound feelings of detachment and loss.

Depressed mood, anxiety, anger, intense shame or guilt feelings, distractibility, irritability, and an exaggerated startle response may continue for years following exposure to trauma. Severely traumatized individuals may experience psychotic symptoms including dissociative symptoms (e.g. difficulty perceiving their body or the environment as real), and auditory or visual hallucinations.

Biological and environmental factors that affect the risk of developing PTSD include genetic susceptibility, the developmental stage when exposure to trauma occurs, culture and socioeconomic issues, and the presence of other mental health problems. The particular symptoms experienced by a traumatized individual probably reflect complex interactions between genes coding for serotonin, norepinephrine and other neurotransmitters, and the timing, severity and frequency of traumatic exposure.

Women, youth, individuals from low-income neighborhoods, and individuals who have pre-existing problems with depressed mood or anxiety are at increased risk of developing PTSD following exposure to trauma. Combat veterans diagnosed with PTSD are at significantly greater risk of committing suicide. A significant percentage of combat veterans diagnosed with PTSD also suffer from traumatic brain injury, making treatment of PTSD symptoms even more difficult.

The enormous personal, social and economic burden of human suffering, treatment costs, disability compensation, and productivity losses related to PTSD are major issues facing American society at this time because of the recent military conflicts in the Middle East. It is estimated that approximately 300,000 active duty or recently discharged U.S. military veterans currently have or will develop PTSD or major depressive disorder as a consequence of those conflicts.

PTSD resulting from violent assault, rape or traumatic exposure to combat is often characterized by severe symptoms that are poorly response to treatment. In fact, as many as one half of all persons diagnosed with PTSD who are treated with prescription medications or psychological therapies do not fully respond.

The majority of individuals diagnosed with PTSD have at least one other mental health problem such as generalized anxiety disorder, panic disorder, phobic disorders, major depressive disorder, obsessive-compulsive disorder, anti-social personality disorder, and alcohol or drug abuse. Medical disorders that frequently occur together with PTSD include cardiovascular disease, arthritis, hypertension and autoimmune disorders. Acute Stress Disorder (ASD) is a less severe variant of PTSD in which all symptoms resolve within one month following exposure to trauma. Roughly one half of individuals who are diagnosed with ASD eventually develop full-blown PTSD.

Taking inventory of your symptoms

This section will help you understand your PTSD symptoms better and determine how severe they are. Let's start by defining what the word *symptom* means. A *symptom is something you experience inside that you can't see. It's a subjective experience of distress that can point to a medical or mental health problem.* When different symptoms occur together, they make up a particular mental health problem or *disorder*.

While many individuals who are diagnosed with PTSD have similar symptoms each person's symptoms are related to their *unique* biological constitution, social and family history and personal circumstances. Symptoms of PTSD can be mild, moderate or severe in intensity depending on how much distress they cause and how much they interfere with your ability to function in day to day activities.

Taking inventory of your PTSD symptoms involves filling in a symptom check-list or answering standardized questions. Going through this process will give you important insights that will help you put together a treatment plan based on your particular symptoms. If you are reading the e-book you can click here to get to psychological assessment tools that you can use to evaluate your anxiety problem and the other mental health problems covered in this series of books. If you are reading the print book you can find on-line psychological assessment tools at http://www.theintegrativementalhealthsolution.com/self-assesment-questionaires.html.

Remember to keep a record of your results so that you can track changes in your PTSD symptoms over time. I encourage you to take inventory frequently in order to find out how well your symptoms are responding to treatment. You can use the results to optimize your current treatment plan or develop a completely new treatment plan.

If you have PTSD and another mental health problem at the same time, I encourage you to complete the self-assessment test for that problem also.

Identifying treatments that make sense for you: evaluating the evidence

This section provides concise reviews of the evidence for a variety of alternative treatments of PTSD. In addition to natural supplements, many other approaches are beneficial for PTSD including virtual reality graded exposure therapy, EEG biofeedback, Chinese medicine, yoga, and meditation.

Natural supplements used to treat PTSD include a multi-nutrient formula, dehydroepiandrosterone (DHEA) and essential fatty acids. The majority of herbals and other natural supplements have few or mild adverse effects when a quality brand is used at the recommended dosage. However, some natural supplements can cause serious side effects when taken at inappropriate high dosages or in combination with certain medications. *Please read the comments on safety before trying any herbal or other natural*

supplement.

The various alternative approaches used to treat PTSD can be divided into 5 categories:

- **Biological treatments** have beneficial effects at the level of one or more well-defined molecular mechanisms. Natural supplements work in this way.

- **Whole body approaches** have general beneficial effects on the body as a whole, improve both physical and mental health and enhance well-being. Exercise and massage are examples of whole-body approaches.

- **Mindfulness and mind-body approaches** are based on concepts from traditional healing aimed at improving the harmony between mind and body. Approaches in this category include awareness training, breathing techniques and mental imagery. While some mindfulness and mind-body approaches are based on a particular spiritual belief system, you do not need to believe in God or have a spiritual orientation in order to benefit from these practices. Yoga, Tai-chi, and transcendental meditation are examples.

- **Treatments based on scientifically verified forms of energy** including electricity, magnetic fields, light and sound have beneficial effects at many levels in the body and brain. Examples include full-spectrum bright light exposure, weak electrical current, EEG biofeedback, and specialized forms of sound therapy.

- **Treatments based on subtle forms of energy** that have not been verified by science such as Reiki, qigong, prayer, Healing Touch and Therapeutic Touch may be beneficial at the level of postulated energetic processes that may play a role in maintaining optimal physical and psychological wellness, and for treating some mental health problems.

Most vitamins, minerals and essential fatty acids are examples of natural supplements that can be safely used without the advice or supervision of a physician or other health care provider. However, some natural supplements derived from plants or other natural products cause potentially serious safety problems and it is important to adhere to recommended dosages when using these supplements and avoid taking them with medications that are known to cause unsafe toxic interactions.

When a natural supplement is known to cause potentially serious adverse effects or toxicities ***important safety warnings are in bold face, underlined and in italics. I encourage you to consult with a knowledgeable health care provider for advice on the safe and appropriate use of any supplement that has potentially serious adverse effects***.

While some people prefer to use a medication or a natural supplement, others benefit from combining a supplement or medication with a whole-body approach, a mind-body practice, or energy work. The treatment plan you decide to use will depend not only on the evidence supporting it but also the amount of time you have to try a particular approach, and your level of motivation.

Meditation, mindfulness training, dance and movement therapy, as well as Tai Chi, yoga, massage and Qigong are beneficial for symptoms of PTSD. There are no safety concerns when using such approaches while taking a natural supplement or a medication. However, in some cases it takes a great deal of time, effort and experience to use a whole-body or mind body or energy therapy properly before you can expect to benefit.

Finally, you may have a better or more rapid response if you consistently try yoga, meditation or Qigong or another approach while taking an appropriate supplement or a medication. Such combined treatment regimens are examples of integrative mental health care, as described above.

Alternative treatments of PTSD

This section reviews the evidence for specific natural supplements, whole-body approaches, mind-body and mindfulness practices, and energy therapies used to treat PTSD. The following information is listed in bullets so that you can compare research evidence and safety information for a variety of treatment choices:

- Name of treatment and category

- How the treatment works (where known)

- Dosages (for natural supplements) or frequency or duration of use (for whole body, mind-body or energy approaches)

- Examples of safe and effective treatment combinations

- Comments about adverse effects and warnings pertaining to the treatment or treatment combinations that may result in potentially unsafe interactions and should be avoided

- Average duration of treatment needed to achieve beneficial results

I use a '3-tier' approach to rate treatments based on the relative strength of evidence.

- **Tier A:** treatments are supported by strong research evidence from rigorously conducted studies or systematic reviews of studies.

- **Tier B:** treatments are also supported by research evidence but not to the same degree as tier A treatments.

- **Tier C:** treatments are supported by weak or inconsistent research findings and may be effective in some cases

Note that treatments under each tier are listed in alphabetical order and not according to the relative level of evidence.

Tier A treatments of PTSD

Please note that at this time no alternative treatments of PTSD are supported by the highest level of research evidence.

Tier B treatments of PTSD

- Chinese medicine

- Dance/movement therapy

- EEG biofeedback training

- Meditation and mindfulness training

- Qigong and Tai Chi

- Virtual reality exposure therapy (VRET)

- Yoga

Chinese medicine

- **Name of treatment and category:** Chinese medicine is a highly evolved system of medicine that includes acupuncture, herbal medicine, energetic massage (also called *tui na*), moxibustion, specialized diets, and qigong.

- **How the treatment works:** The techniques used in Chinese medicine work in many different ways. According to Chinese medical theory acupuncture, herbals and other treatments *re-balance* the body's vital energy resulting in improved health. Research findings show that acupuncture and other techniques used in Chinese medicine have beneficial effects at many levels in the body and brain, including changes in the levels of neurotransmitters involved in the response to chronic stress. Regular acupuncture may decrease the severity of so-called *core symptoms* of PTSD as well as symptoms that frequently occur in traumatized refugees, torture survivors and combat veterans such as headaches, anxiety, fatigue, sleep disturbances, depression and chronic pain.

- **Dosages (for natural supplements) or frequency of use (for whole body, mind-body or energy approaches):** Treatments for PTSD recommended by a Chinese medical practitioner depend on the findings of an energetic assessment based on a specialized reading of the pulse. Each person has a unique *energetic profile* that translates into individualized treatment recommendations for different people even when outward symptoms of trauma are similar.

- **Examples of safe and effective treatment combinations:** Acupuncture, energetic massage, moxibustion, dietary changes and Qigong may be safely combined with modalities from all other treatment categories. Certain Chinese herbal formulas may be safely combined with prescription medications enhancing their effectiveness against symptoms of PTSD and in some cases permitting reductions in medication dosages.

- **Comments about adverse effects and warnings pertaining to treatment combinations that may result in potentially unsafe interactions and should be avoided:** Acupuncture is generally safe when practiced by a qualified Chinese medical practitioner. Worsening of PTSD symptoms (i.e. re-traumatization) following acupuncture has not been reported. Acupuncture may cause minor bruising, bleeding or pain. Chinese herbal formulas are generally safe when taken at recommended dosages under the supervision of a qualified Chinese medical practitioner. *Caution: taking certain Chinese herbals may cause serious adverse effects when taken alone or in combination with certain prescription medications. Therefore, when considering taking Chinese herbal medicines for PTSD or any other medical or mental health problem it is always preferable to work with a knowledgeable and highly experienced Chinese medical practitioner.*

- **Average duration of treatment needed to achieve beneficial results:** Some individuals experience significant decreases in the severity of PTSD symptoms after several weeks of Chinese medical treatments under the supervision of an experienced and well-trained practitioner.

Dance/movement therapy

- **Name of treatment and category:** Dance/movement therapy combines a whole-body approach with elements of cognitive psychotherapy.

- **How the treatment works:** Dance/movement therapy increases body awareness and helps individuals process the cognitive and psychological consequences of trauma resulting in improved coping with stressful situations. Dance/movement therapy may decrease the severity of intrusive memories, anxiety and aggression which are common symptoms in torture survivors.

- **Dosages (for natural supplements) or frequency of use (for whole body, mind-body or energy approaches):** Some torture survivors who participate in weekly 1 hour or longer sessions of dance/movement therapy experience significant decreases in arousal, anxiety, flashbacks and other symptoms of PTSD.

- **Examples of safe and effective treatment combinations:** Dance/movement therapy may be safely combined with other treatment categories.

- **Comments about adverse effects and warnings pertaining to treatment combinations that may result in potentially unsafe interactions and should be avoided:** *Caution: Some trauma survivors experience temporary worsening of PTSD symptoms with dance/movement therapy.*

- **Average duration of treatment needed to achieve beneficial results:** Some individuals experience significant decreases in the severity of PTSD symptoms after several weeks of dance/movement therapy.

EEG biofeedback (also called neurofeedback or neurotherapy)

- **Name of treatment and category:** EEG biofeedback is a scientifically validated energy therapy in which pre-selected features of brain electrical activity are modified during an interactive game.

- **How the treatment works:** When engaged in EEG biofeedback the individual is rewarded and allowed to advance to the next position in a game when specific changes in brain activity take place showing that a calmer or more focused mental state has been achieved. Continued training in select brainwave frequencies increases the individual's ability to achieve a target state of brain activity corresponding to reduced anxiety. EEG biofeedback is widely used to treat Attention Deficit

Hyperactivity Disorder (ADHD) and anxiety disorders in children and adults.

- **Dosages (for natural supplements) or frequency of use (for whole body, mind-body or energy approaches):** EEG biofeedback therapy is administered by a psychotherapist certified in this technique. Sessions may last 30 minutes or longer and individuals diagnosed with PTSD may receive 1 to 3 sessions weekly. Recent research findings suggest that EEG biofeedback training at very low frequencies (so-called *infra-low* frequencies of less than one cycle per second) may significantly decrease the severity of PTSD symptoms in combat veterans.

- **Examples of safe and effective treatment combinations:** EEG biofeedback training may be safely combined with other treatment categories. Some EEG biofeedback therapists recommend discontinuing or reducing dosages of prescription medications before starting training in the belief that doing so may enhance the effectiveness of EEG biofeedback.

- **Comments about adverse effects and warnings pertaining to treatment combinations that may result in potentially unsafe interactions and should be avoided:** none.

- **Average duration of treatment needed to achieve beneficial results:** Some combat veterans experience moderate to significant decreases in PTSD symptom severity after 10 to 20 sessions of EEG biofeedback.

Meditation and mindfulness training

- **Name of treatment and category:** Different styles of meditation including transcendental meditation, Vipassana (also called *insight*) meditation and others, belong to the general category of mindfulness practices.

- **How the treatment works:** The regular practice of meditation *before* exposure to trauma may reduce the risk of developing PTSD following trauma and lessen the severity of symptoms in individuals diagnosed with chronic PTSD. Meditation and other mindfulness practices may give traumatized individuals greater control over intrusive thoughts and disturbing memories while helping them shift their attention from fearful memories to problem solving in the present resulting in improved coping in stressful situations. A style of meditation that emphasizes the development of compassion and empathy (Vipassana) may decrease negative emotions and reactivity to stressful circumstances in individuals diagnosed with PTSD. Group meditation practice increases social connections and improves resilience in traumatized individuals.

- **Dosages (for natural supplements) or frequency of use (for whole body, mind-body or energy approaches):** Group meditation programs addressing trauma often take place weekly and typical sessions last 1 to 2 hours. In addition to group practice many individuals diagnosed with PTSD benefit from a daily individual meditation practice. Regular meditation practice is beneficial for symptoms of anxiety and depressed mood which frequently occur together with PTSD.

- **Examples of safe and effective treatment combinations:** Meditation and other mindfulness training approaches may be safely combined with modalities in other treatment categories.

- **Comments about adverse effects and warnings pertaining to treatment combinations that may result in potentially unsafe interactions and should be avoided:** *Caution: some individuals diagnosed with PTSD experience intense anxiety, panic attacks or flashbacks when meditating or practicing relaxation.*

- **Average duration of treatment needed to achieve beneficial results:** Some individuals diagnosed with PTSD experience significant decreases in the severity of their symptoms after several weeks of regular meditation practice.

Qigong and Tai Chi

- **Name of treatment and category:** Tai chi and Qigong are energetic approaches used in Chinese medicine that have not been scientifically validated.

- **How the treatment works:** The regular practice of tai chi or qigong enhances self-awareness of the body and provides beneficial calming effects that improve general well-being and may lessen the severity of the negative psychological and physical consequences of torture in refugees and traumatic experiences in combat veterans. Both approaches may help decrease symptoms of anxiety, disturbed sleep, depressed mood and dissociation which frequently occur in individuals diagnosed with PTSD.

- **Dosages (for natural supplements) or frequency of use (for whole body, mind-body or energy approaches):** Tai chi and qigong may be practiced individually or in a group under the supervision of a knowledgeable instructor. Many individuals develop their own daily practice in the context of regular weekly groups.

- **Examples of safe and effective treatment combinations:** Tai chi and qigong may be safely combined with other approaches.

- **Comments about adverse effects and warnings pertaining to treatment combinations that may result in potentially unsafe interactions and should be avoided:** Tai chi and qigong are very low-impact practices with negligible risk of physical injury. *Caution: so-called activating tai chi or qigong routines may cause temporary worsening of the* *psychological consequences of trauma thus it is advisable to practice tai chi or qigong under the guidance of an instructor who has experience working with trauma.*

- **Average duration of treatment needed to achieve beneficial results:** Some individuals experience significant and sustained decreases in the severity of PTSD symptoms after several weeks of regular tai chi or qigong practice.

Virtual reality graded exposure therapy (VRGET)

- **Name of treatment and category:** VRGET is a technology-based exposure therapy that uses advanced computer technology.

- **How the treatment works:** VRGET uses computer graphics, 3D displays and multi-sensory feedback to create a feeling of immersion in a computer-generated world. Immersion in this virtual world makes you feel like you are in a dangerous situation and causes intense anxiety which gradually lessens after several sessions. A therapist may be present to guide the individual undergoing VRGET in relaxation exercises such as deep breathing or guided imagery. VRGET administered prior to exposure to trauma (e.g. combat) may be an effective intervention for preventing PTSD, or reducing the severity of PTSD symptoms that develop after trauma.

- **Dosages (for natural supplements) or frequency of use (for whole body, mind-body or energy approaches):** VRGET sessions typically last between 30 and 45 minutes and are administered weekly or more often.

- **Examples of safe and effective treatment combinations:** Combining VRGET with EEG biofeedback or heart-rate variability (HRV) biofeedback may be a more effective treatment of PTSD than VRGET alone. Combining VRGET with D-cycloserine may be more effective and yield more rapid beneficial results than VRGET alone.

- **Comments about adverse effects and warnings pertaining to treatment combinations that may result in potentially unsafe interactions and should be avoided:** VRGET is generally safe when used appropriately under the supervision of a therapist trained in this technique. Some individuals experience mild feelings of temporary disorientation, nausea, dizziness, headache or blurred vision. "Simulator sleepiness" is an infrequent adverse effect of VRGET characterized by transient feelings of intense fatigue. *__Caution: there are rare reports of VRGET triggering migraine headaches, seizures, or gait abnormalities. Individuals who have these medical problems should consider using VRGET only after giving informed consent and only under close medical supervision.__*

- **Average duration of treatment needed to achieve beneficial results:** Many individuals diagnosed with PTSD experience significant and sustained decreases in the severity of their symptoms after 4 to 10 VRGET sessions administered over a period of several days or weeks.

Yoga

- **Name of treatment and category:** Yoga is a mind-body approach.

- **How the treatment works:** Yoga postures (asanas) and specialized breathing techniques (pranayamas) have general calming effects on the body and mind. The regular practice of yoga may have beneficial effects on the electrical activity of the brain and neurotransmitters resulting in decreased anxiety, improved mood, improved sleep, enhanced capacity to cope with stress, and generally improved quality of life.

- **Dosages (for natural supplements) or frequency of use (for whole body, mind-body or energy approaches):** Yoga practice can be done individually or in a supervised group setting. Typical yoga sessions last 30 minutes to one hour depending on the style of yoga and the experience level of the practitioner.

- **Examples of safe and effective treatment combinations:** Yoga may be safely used in combination with other approaches.

- **Comments about adverse effects and warnings pertaining to treatment combinations that may result in potentially unsafe interactions and should be avoided:** Yoga is generally safe when practiced under the guidance of a qualified yoga instructor. _**Caution: individuals with chronic pain conditions or other physical limitations should consult with a health care provider before starting a rigorous yoga practice. Caution: certain yoga postures (asanas) may**_ *increase feelings of vulnerability in torture survivors. Strenuous yoga poses may remind trauma survivors of previous traumatic experiences resulting in the temporary worsening of PTSD symptoms.*

- **Average duration of treatment needed to achieve beneficial results:** Many trauma survivors experience significant reductions in PTSD symptoms after several weeks of regular yoga practice.

Tier C approaches used to prevent or treat PTSD

- Binaural sound

- Cardiac coherence training

- Dehydroepiandrosterone (DHEA)

- Energy healing approaches (Thought-field therapy (TFT), emotional freedom technique (EFT) and others)

- Lucid dreaming training

- Massage

- Multi-nutrient formula

- Music

- Omega-3 essential fatty acids

- Reiki

- Spirituality and religion

Binaural sound

- **Name of treatment and category:** The binaural 'beat' is the sound frequency that is perceived when sounds of different frequencies are delivered to the left and right ears.

- **How the treatment works:** Psychological benefits of listening to binaural beats include reduced anxiety, improved focusing, enhanced concentration and improved mood. 'Reconsolidation Enhancement by Stimulation of Emotional Triggers' (RESET) is a specialized technique that employs binaural beats to treat symptoms of PTSD. listening to certain binaural beats is believed to rebalance the sympathetic and parasympathetic nervous systems resulting decoupling of brain regions involved in linking intense emotions to long-term memories. The goal of therapy is to diminish the emotional intensity of memories of trauma and (when successful) to completely remove memories of trauma.

- **Dosages (for natural supplements) or frequency of use (for whole body, mind-body or energy approaches):** Sham-controlled trials on RESET therapy using binaural sounds have not been done at the time of writing (September, 2019). Findings of a few case reports suggest that listening to certain binaural sound frequencies for several minutes at a time, a few times weekly may significantly reduce the emotional intensity of memories of trauma, and help traumatized individuals to 'let go of' memories of trauma.

- **Examples of safe and effective treatment combinations:** Binaural sounds may be safely used in combination with other conventional or CAM approaches.

- **Comments about adverse effects and warnings pertaining to treatment combinations that may result in potentially unsafe interactions and should be avoided:** none

- **Average duration of treatment needed to achieve beneficial results:** Some veterans have reported significant reductions in the severity of PTSD symptoms after only a few brief sessions of RESET therapy using binaural sound.

Cardiac coherence training

- **Name of treatment and category:** Cardiac coherence training is a type of biofeedback that uses information about heart rate variability (HRV) to train individuals in reducing their anxiety or improving their ability to focus.

- **How the treatment works:** Abnormalities in HRV are associated with problems in attention and short-term memory in combat veterans diagnosed with PTSD. Limited research findings suggest that cardiac coherence training may be as effective as prescription medications for decreasing PTSD symptoms in some combat veterans.

- **Dosages (for natural supplements) or frequency of use (for whole body, mind-body or energy approaches):** There is no agreement on the optimal frequency or total number of cardiac coherence training sessions for individuals diagnosed with PTSD however many individuals benefit from weekly sessions 30 minutes or longer.

- **Examples of safe and effective treatment combinations:** Cardiac coherence training may be safely used with other treatment approaches. Combining HRV biofeedback with relaxation training may improve attention and short-term memory in individuals diagnosed with PTSD.

- **Comments about adverse effects and warnings pertaining to treatment combinations that may result in potentially unsafe interactions and should be avoided:** none

- **Average duration of treatment needed to achieve beneficial results:** Some combat veterans experience significant reductions in the severity of PTSD symptoms after 2 to 4 weeks of regular HRV biofeedback training.

Dehydroepiandrosterone (DHEA)

- **Name of treatment and category:** DHEA is naturally present in the body and is used to make several hormones that play important roles in the body and brain. The related molecule 7-keto-DHEA may be more effective than DHEA.

- **How the treatment works:** DHEA may protect the brain from the negative effects of stress.

- **Dosages (for natural products) or frequency of use (for somatic, mind-body or energy approaches):** DHEA (especially in the form 7-keto-DHEA) taken at doses between 25 and 100mg/day may decrease PTSD symptoms that do not improve with prescription medications, such as numbing, re-experiencing and hyper-arousal.

- **Examples of safe and effective treatment combinations:** DHEA may be safely combined with most natural products and prescription medications. DHEA may have beneficial add-on mood-elevating effects when taken together with an antidepressant.

- **Comments about adverse effects and warnings pertaining to treatment combinations that may result in potentially unsafe interactions and should be avoided:** DHEA is generally safe when taken at recommended dosages. *Caution: women should avoid taking DHEA if there is a history of estrogen receptor positive breast cancer however the 7-keto-DHEA form is probably safe in this population. Men should avoid taking DHEA if they have a history of prostate cancer or an elevated PSA.*

- **Average duration of treatment needed to achieve beneficial results:** Some individuals diagnosed with PTSD experience significant decreases in the severity of their symptoms after taking 7-keto-DHEA 25mg/day for several days.

Energy healing

- **Name of treatment and category:** Energy healing approaches have not been scientifically validated. Different energy healing approaches used to treat PTSD include Healing touch (HT), Therapeutic touch (TT), energy psychology, thought-field therapy (TFT), emotional freedom technique (EFT) and specialized spiritual methods in Ayurveda, Tibetan medicine, and shamanic ritual healing. *Reiki is reviewed under a separate entry.*

- **How the treatment works:** The mechanisms underlying energy healing are poorly understood but may involve psychological, biological and possibly so-called *subtle* energetic processes related to quantum mechanics. Some energy healing approaches are administered by certified practitioners whereas EFT, TFT and other energy healing approaches involve simple techniques and can be self-administered after brief training.

- **Dosages (for natural supplements) or frequency of use (for whole body, mind-body or energy approaches):** Healing touch, emotional freedom technique and other energy healing approaches administered or self-administered twice weekly may significantly decrease the severity of PTSD symptoms.

- **Examples of safe and effective treatment combinations:** Energy healing approaches may be safely used in conjunction with other approaches.

- **Comments about adverse effects and warnings pertaining to treatment combinations that may result in potentially unsafe interactions and should be avoided:** none

- **Average duration of treatment needed to achieve beneficial results:** Some individuals experience significant decreases in the severity of PTSD symptoms after several weeks of regular treatment with energy healing.

Lucid dreaming training

- **Name of treatment and category:** Lucid dreaming is a unique state of consciousness in which an individual is self-aware while dreaming, and able to change or control dream content.

- **How the treatment works:** Lucid dreaming techniques such as "dialoging with" or "physically embracing" dream characters may reduce feelings of helplessness and terror as the individual learns that he or she can control frightening images or experiences associated with trauma. Training in lucid dreaming may reduce the severity and frequency of nightmares in individuals diagnosed with PTSD however other symptoms of PTSD may remain unchanged.

- **Dosages (for natural supplements) or frequency of use (for whole body, mind-body or energy approaches):** Training in lucid dreaming methods typically involves 4 to 6 weeks of daily dream journaling and weekly sessions for training in specific lucid dream-induction techniques focusing on insights related to recurrent nightmares.

- **Examples of safe and effective treatment combinations:** Training in lucid dreaming methods may be safely combined with other approaches.

- **Comments about adverse effects and warnings pertaining to treatment combinations that may result in potentially unsafe interactions and should be avoided:** none.

- **Average duration of treatment needed to achieve beneficial results:** Some individuals diagnosed with PTSD are able to achieve lucidity and develop skill at reducing the frequency of recurring nightmares after participating in a 4 to 6-week program in lucid dreaming training (above).

Massage therapy

- **Name of treatment and category:** massage therapy is a whole-body approach.

- **How the treatment works:** Regular massage relaxes the body and increases brain levels of serotonin and dopamine resulting in general calming effects. Regular massage may reduce muscle tension, decrease symptoms of dissociation and increase body awareness in individuals diagnosed with PTSD. Regular massage may decrease symptoms of depression and anxiety which frequently accompany PTSD.

- **Dosages (for natural supplements) or frequency of use (for whole body, mind-body or energy approaches):** Some individuals diagnosed with PTSD benefit from light to moderate pressure massage administered in weekly 30-minute sessions. There is no agreement on the optimal duration of a massage or the optimal interval between treatments.

- **Examples of safe and effective treatment combinations:** Massage therapy may be safely combined with other approaches.

- **Comments about adverse effects and warnings pertaining to treatment combinations that may result in potentially unsafe interactions and should be avoided:** Massage is generally safe when administered by a qualified massage therapist. *Caution: Survivors of trauma may experience reactivation of latent PTSD symptoms such as intense feelings of anxiety or flashbacks during massage or other body-centered therapies.*

- **Average duration of treatment needed to achieve beneficial results:** Some individuals diagnosed with PTSD experience decreases in symptom severity after several weeks of regular massage.

Multi-nutrient formulas

- **Name of treatment and category:** Multi-nutrient formulas containing vitamins, minerals, amino acids and other natural supplements are used as biological treatments of different medical and mental health problems.

- **How the treatment works:** Natural substances in multi-nutrient formulas are believed to make up for dietary deficiencies or genetic problems that result in greater susceptibility to stress. Taking a multi-nutrient formula on a regular basis before exposure to trauma may increase emotional resilience and reduce the severity of PTSD symptoms following trauma.

- **Dosages (for natural supplements) or frequency of use (for whole body, mind-body or energy approaches):** The recommended daily dosage varies depending on the particular multi-nutrient formula that is being used and whether prescription medications are being used concurrently. Taking 4 to 8 capsules daily of one proprietary multi-nutrient formula (EMPowerPlus™) may decrease the intensity of stress and anxiety that take place in response to trauma and may be as effective as prescription medications and other conventional pharmacologic or psychotherapeutic treatments of PTSD. Taking 4 capsules daily of the above proprietary formula may be as effective as taking 8 capsules/day.

- **Examples of safe and effective treatment combinations:** Some individuals who take a multi-nutrient formula and a prescription mood stabilizer are able to lower the dosage of their prescription medication or stop taking it without experiencing worsening in PTSD symptoms.

- **Comments about adverse effects and warnings pertaining to treatment combinations that may result in potentially unsafe interactions and should be avoided:** Most multi-nutrient formulas are well tolerated however some individuals who take nutrient formulas experience mild temporary adverse effects such as nausea and diarrhea. _**Caution: Interactions between nutrient formulas and prescription medications are potentially dangerous. Anyone considering combining a multi-nutrient formula and a prescription medication should do so under the supervision of a qualified health care provider who is knowledgeable about the specific multi-nutrient formula being considered.**_

• **Average duration of treatment needed to achieve beneficial results:** The optimal duration of treatment has not been clearly established and is probably related to symptom severity and the active constituents and dosage of a multi-nutrient formula being taken. Some individuals diagnosed with PTSD who take multi-nutrient formulas report significant decreases in general stress level over time, as well as reduction in the symptoms of anxiety, avoidance and arousal that frequently occur together with PTSD.

Music

- **Name of treatment and category:** Music and sound are scientifically validated energy techniques used to treat physical and mental health problems in many cultures.

- **How the treatment works:** Listening to music or rhythmic sounds has general calming effects on the brain. Listening to music on a long-term basis may change brain electrical activity or neurotransmitter levels resulting in decreased anxiety and improved mood. Participation in a drumming circle or other culturally appropriate musically oriented group increases feelings of community participation and trust which are often damaged following trauma.

- **Dosages (for natural supplements) or frequency of use (for whole body, mind-body or energy approaches):** Some individuals who participate in weekly or more frequent music therapy, listen to soothing music on a regular basis, use a singing bowl, or engage in a drumming circle or other musically oriented group, experience significant and sustained decreases in the severity of PTSD symptoms.

- **Examples of safe and effective treatment combinations:** Listening to music, formal music therapy or participation in a drumming circle or other musical support group may be safely combined with other approaches.

- **Comments about adverse effects and warnings pertaining to treatment combinations that may result in potentially unsafe interactions and should be avoided:** *Caution: very rare cases of loud sounds evoking a startle response or triggering flashbacks have been reported. The choice of music or sound should be selected with this in mind.*

- **Average duration of treatment needed to achieve beneficial results:** Some trauma survivors experience sustained decreases in PTSD symptoms after several weeks of regular exposure to soothing music or rhythmic sound. Beneficial effects on PTSD are equivalent when this approach is used in a group setting or done privately by single individuals.

Omega-3 essential fatty acids

- **Name of treatment and category:** Omega-3 essential fatty acids occur naturally in many foods including algae, barley and some fishes. The two omega-3s: docosahexanoic acid (DHA) and ecosapentanoic acid (EPA) are used as biological treatments of different medical and mental health problems.

- **How the treatment works:** Omega-3 fatty acids play many essential roles in the body and brain. Taking an omega-3 supplement may be helpful for both preventing and treating PTSD. This is probably related to the fact that omega-3s promote growth in an area of the brain (i.e. the hippocampus) involved in extinguishing memories of trauma thus decreasing *some* symptoms of PTSD.

- **Dosages (for natural supplements) or frequency of use (for whole body, mind-body or energy approaches):** Taking a mixture of omega-3s consisting of DHA (1500mg/day) and EPA (approx. 150mg/day) on an on-going basis *before trauma* may decrease the risk of developing PTSD in the event of subsequent exposure to trauma. Taking the same dosage of omega-3s starting soon after trauma may decrease the severity of PTSD symptoms.

- **Examples of safe and effective treatment combinations:** Omega-3s may be safely combined with other natural products and most prescription medications. Omega-3s may improve the effectiveness of SSRIs and other antidepressant medications widely used to treat PTSD symptoms.

- **Comments about adverse effects and warnings pertaining to treatment combinations that may result in potentially unsafe interactions and should be avoided:** Omega-3s are generally safe and sometimes have mild adverse effects including fishy taste and nausea. *__Caution: high dosages of omega-3s may increase the risk of bleeding and should not be taken together with aspirin or other medications that affect bleeding time.__*

- **Average duration of treatment needed to achieve beneficial results:** The optimal duration for taking omega-3s for preventing or treating PTSD has not been established. Some individuals who take omega-3s (see above dosages) for several weeks prior to a traumatic event may be less likely to develop PTSD if they subsequently exposed to trauma. Some individuals who start taking omega-3s soon after being exposed to trauma may be less likely to develop PTSD.

Reiki

- **Name of treatment and category:** Reiki is an energy therapy dating to early 20th century Japan that has not been scientifically validated.

- **How the treatment works:** During Reiki therapy so-called *universal healing energy* is directed through the hands of a trained practitioner into a patient with the intention of unblocking vital energy resulting in beneficial changes in physical or mental health. Reiki therapy may be administered in the absence of physical contact or through light touch. Research studies suggest that Reiki may decrease the severity of anxiety, depressed mood and chronic pain which often occur together with PTSD in trauma survivors.

- **Dosages (for natural supplements) or frequency of use (for whole body, mind-body or energy approaches):** Many individuals benefit from weekly Reiki therapy lasting 1 to 1 ½ hours. There is no consensus among Reiki practitioners on an optimal frequency or length of Reiki sessions for individuals diagnosed with PTSD.

- **Examples of safe and effective treatment combinations:** Reiki may be safely combined with other approaches.

- **Comments about adverse effects and warnings pertaining to treatment combinations that may result in potentially unsafe interactions and should be avoided:** none.

- **Average duration of treatment needed to achieve beneficial results:** Some individuals experience decreases in the severity of PTSD symptoms after several weeks of regular Reiki therapy.

Spirituality and religion

- **Name of treatment and category:** Spiritual and religious practices do not belong to a particular category and incorporate elements of mindfulness and energy healing approaches.

- **How the treatment works:** Spiritual and religious beliefs and practices provide important insights and a framework of social support that help traumatized individuals function better in society and cope with stress more effectively. The social and psychological benefits of belonging to a spiritual or religious group may decrease the severity of some PTSD symptoms.

- **Dosages (for natural supplements) or frequency of use (for whole body, mind-body or energy approaches):** Some traumatized individuals who follow a spiritual or religious practice or participate in regular support groups with a spiritual theme function better and experience fewer PTSD symptoms compared to individuals who are not religiously or spiritually oriented.

- **Examples of safe and effective treatment combinations:** Other treatments may be safely combined with spiritual or religious practices.

- **Comments about adverse effects and warnings pertaining to treatment combinations that may result in potentially unsafe interactions and should be avoided:** none

- **Average duration of treatment needed to achieve beneficial results:** Religious or spiritual beliefs and practices are integral parts of daily life for many people. Traumatized individuals often benefit from long-term participation in group religious practices, individual spiritual practices, or a weekly support group with a spiritual focus.

Before starting treatment

The treatment or treatment combination you decide to try after reading this book will be based on your history, symptoms, preferences and circumstances. As you learn how to think about your mental health care in a more holistic way using the information and methods in this book you will discover more effective approaches for taking care of your PTSD symptoms.

Before starting one or more of the above treatments I encourage you to finish reading this entire book to make sure you know how to develop a plan that is *right for you*. If you have another mental health problem in addition to PTSD, I encourage you to read the book in the series on that condition or find another reliable source of information before starting any new treatment.

Deciding on a treatment plan that is *right for you*

General considerations

Now that you've learned about a variety of alternative treatment choices for PTSD the next step is to decide on treatments that address your particular symptoms keeping in mind treatment choices that are available where you live and within your budget.

As I mentioned earlier, because your history and your symptoms are *unique,* the best treatment plan for you may be different from the best treatment plan for someone else. In other words, *there is no single best treatment for everyone who has PTSD.* I've created a simple method that will help you put together a treatment plan addressing your particular symptoms.

The best treatment plan *for you* is based on:

- research evidence

- your response to treatments you've already tried

- your personal preferences

- treatments that are available where you live

- what you can afford

Do you have a medical problem that may be making your PTSD symptoms worse or interfering with treatment?

At the beginning of this book I described some medical problems that sometimes occur together with PTSD including cardiovascular disease, arthritis, hypertension and autoimmune disorders. When an underlying medical problem is diagnosed and properly treated, symptoms of PTSD may improve rapidly, and you may start to respond better to the treatment you've been taking until now without benefit.

Depressed mood, anxiety disorders, and substance abuse often occur together with PTSD. Both of these mental health problems can worsen PTSD symptoms and interfere with response to treatment. Many combat veterans diagnosed with PTSD have a history of traumatic brain injury. This condition, called *complex trauma*, can exacerbate symptoms of PTSD and make it more difficult to respond to treatment. If you are a combat veteran with complex trauma, I strongly encourage you to consult with a psychiatrist at the VA where you receive care, or another mental health care provider who has experience treating this challenging condition.

First steps

This section will guide you through the steps needed to develop a treatment plan that is appropriate for you whether you have moderate or severe PTSD symptoms. The first step is deciding on an appropriate treatment plan involves identifying one or more treatments that you are *open to* trying.

Recall that no currently available alternative treatments are supported by the highest level of evidence (i.e., none are in tier A). When developing a treatment plan, you probably have a better chance of *feeling better* and *staying well* if you try at least one tier B treatment. This is especially true if you have severe symptoms that are impairing your ability to function at work, in school or in a relationship. Examples of Tier B treatments for PTSD include mindfulness meditation, yoga, EEG biofeedback training and virtual reality graded exposure therapy (VRGET).

If you are experiencing severe PTSD symptoms you may need *to take a medication under the supervision of a psychiatrist.* Even if you need to take a medication, you may benefit from taking one or more natural supplements (i.e., assuming it is safe to do so) or trying other approaches described in this book. Although not supported by strong research findings, natural supplements such as DHEA, multi-nutrient formulas and omega-3 fatty acids are sometimes beneficial, and may be safely combined with psychotropic medications. In addition to natural supplements, other alternative approaches that sometimes help ameliorate PTSD symptoms include a regular mindfulness practice, music therapy, cardiac coherence training, dance therapy, yoga, Qigong, Tai Chi and Reiki.

If you are already taking a psychotropic medication for your PTSD symptoms, I strongly encourage you to *consult with a psychiatrist before starting any new treatment.*

Deciding on a treatment plan that is *right for you*

Since you've gotten this far, I am assuming that your PTSD symptoms *aren't severe* enough to require an emergency room visit or hospitalization. I'm also assuming that if you have been recently hospitalized for severe symptoms of PTSD or another serious mental health problem, you've been discharged, and you are feeling and functioning better now. I am also assuming that *you don't have a medical problem* that is *making your PTSD symptoms worse.* If these things describe your situation, you're ready to start working on a holistic treatment plan that addresses your PTSD symptoms keeping in mind treatments that are available where you live and within your budget.

Finally, if you are experiencing severe PTSD symptoms that are impairing your ability to function, I encourage you to consult with a psychiatrist before starting any new treatment including those discussed in this book.

Taking care of moderately severe symptoms of PTSD

If you have long-standing symptoms of PTSD that are moderately severe and do not impair your ability to function day to day, you may benefit from a regular mindfulness practice, increased physical activity and improved sleep. In addition to such life style changes, some natural supplements and mind-body approaches can help reduce the severity of your PTSD symptoms. For example, the regular practice of mindfulness meditation, yoga, tai chi or qigong can help.

Even if you have already tried many tier B approaches without success, you may benefit from tier C approaches. For example, tier C treatments such as a multi-nutrient formula, DHEA, omega-3 fatty acids, training in lucid dreaming, energy healing approaches, regular massage, or omega-3 fatty acids may reduce the severity of your PTSD symptoms, in some cases allowing you to reduce the dose of a medication and possibly even discontinuing it.

Before trying a Tier C approach, I encourage you to first carefully review the detailed descriptions of Tier B treatments you've already tried to be sure you've used them in ways that *would be expected to be* effective. For example, some people who have used a particular natural supplement with disappointing results find out only later that they had been taking a dosage that was too low, stopped taking it before it had enough time to work, or were not using a quality brand.

I encourage you to check the on-line resources at the end of this book to compare different brands of the natural supplement you've already tried. This will help you find out whether you were taking a quality brand of the supplement at a dose that *would be expected to work*.

If it turns out you didn't take a natural supplement at the recommended dosage or you used a brand of uncertain quality, I

encourage you to try it again, this time taking a quality brand at the recommended dosage and for the recommended duration.

The above reasoning applies equally to treatments other than natural supplements. For example, if you previously used a mind-body therapy or an energy therapy to treat symptoms of PTSD, with disappointing results, I encourage you to check the information in the treatment summaries before concluding that the mind-body or energy treatment you previously tried is ineffective.

If you were not working with an experienced practitioner when you previously tried a mind-body, mindfulness or energetic treatment approach, you *may not have used the most effective technique or tried the approach for an amount of time that would be expected to improve your PTSD symptoms.* I encourage you to *re-evaluate the way you previously used the mindfulness, mind-body practice or energy therapy to find out whether you were doing so in a way and for a duration that would be expected to be beneficial.*

Remember, the treatment or treatments you decide to try after reading this book or other books in the series provide only a *starting place* for a treatment plan that *is right for you.*

Other considerations

In addition to alternative treatment preferences you have after reading this book, I encourage you to remain open to other approaches before deciding on a final treatment plan. If you have already tried several different treatments one at a time, you may have more success trying two or more approaches at the same time starting with treatments in Tier B. This strategy can be especially helpful if:

- a Tier B treatment you've previously tried was helpful but caused side effects and you had to stop using it

- There is evidence that combining a particular Tier B treatment with a medication or particular Tier C treatment will work better than taking a Tier B treatment alone

- a preferred Tier B treatment is unavailable where you live or too expensive

When to manage your PTSD symptoms on your own and when to seek advice from a psychiatrist or other mental healthcare provider

After you have identified approaches you would like to try, the next step involves deciding whether to follow your treatment plan on your own or see a psychiatrist or other mental healthcare provider for expert advice and guidance. The information included under the various treatments will help you decide between self-care and working with an experienced provider.

I encourage you to consult with a psychiatrist if you are experiencing severe symptoms of PTSD or *if you are considering taking any natural supplement together with a medication.*

Below I've listed some important points that will help you find an experienced alternative healthcare practitioner:

- A psychiatrist or other mental health care provider you already know can often help you find an experienced practitioner of an alternative therapy that interests you. If you don't already have a relationship with a psychiatrist or other mental healthcare provider, you can probably get helpful information about local alternative healthcare practitioners from a clinic near you. Many alternative healthcare practitioners are members of a professional association of certified practitioners in their field. A representative of the appropriate professional association—whether it is on Chinese medicine, EEG biofeedback, yoga, energy medicine, or any another healing discipline—can probably recommend one or more practitioners near you.

- Once you've identified an experienced alternative practitioner, I encourage you to learn everything you can about their background, including their education, training, licensing, and advanced certifications. Different professional groups and different countries impose a wide variety of requirements on alternative health care practitioners in terms of training and standards of practice. The most important thing is to identify a practitioner who has a good reputation among his or her colleagues and has extensive experience working with PTSD.

- The next step involves finding out what the treatment costs. I am assuming that many readers have health insurance which may cover at least part of the cost of treatment. Not checking on cost and insurance issues before starting treatment can result in an expensive and brief encounter with even the most qualified practitioner, and leave you feeling disappointed and frustrated with fewer resources remaining to help you get the care you need.

- At the first session it is important to provide your new health care provider with a complete list of treatments you've already tried including those that did not work or caused side effects. Your new provider will use this information to identify approaches that are more likely to be beneficial while minimizing the risk of side effects.

- Be sure to tell your new health care provider *and all other providers*, about changes in your symptoms, any new medical problems, and new treatments that you decide to try. Good communication between yourself and your health care providers will ensure they have the information they need to give you the best possible care.

Safety is *always* the *Number 1* priority

Safety is the *single most important consideration* when you are thinking of starting any new treatment—including a medication, a natural supplement—or a combination of two or more treatments. Though serious safety problems are uncommon, *combinations of certain supplements and medications can result in toxic interactions that may be dangerous and in rare cases life-threatening.*

In the treatment summaries I list known safety concerns for natural supplements when taken alone or with medications. There is a great deal to know about safety that I cannot adequately cover in this short book. *Before taking any natural supplement together with a medication I encourage you to check the on-line resources at the end of this book to find out whether the particular combination you are considering is both effective and safe.*

Making changes along the way: re-evaluating your treatment plan and making it better

This section will help you find out how well your treatment plan is working and know what to do if it is not helping. You will learn when to continue your current treatment plan, change it, or stop it all together.

If you are not functioning better *after following your initial treatment plan for the suggested amount of time* it is important re-evaluate what you are doing and consider making changes. If you have a medical problem that may be making your PTSD symptoms worse or interfering with the treatment(s) you are using, I encourage you to see a psychiatrist or other medically trained provider to find out whether your medical problem requires treatment and to make sure it is not making your PTSD symptoms worse or interfering with the beneficial effects of treatment.

If your treatment plan involves taking a natural supplement or using another approach supported by solid evidence, and you've followed your plan for the *amount of time that is usually needed to achieve beneficial results but you are not feeling and functioning better*, you should consider:

- Increasing the dosage of a natural supplement or medication

- Finding a higher quality brand of a natural supplement or medication

- Increasing the frequency of a whole-body, mind-body or energy therapy

- Adding another approach to your existing treatment plan

- Switching to an entirely new treatment plan

- Stopping treatment all together

If you've already tried several approaches in tier B but without success, you may benefit from combining two tier B treatments or treatments from tiers B and C—*assuming it is safe to do so.*

Although tier C treatments for PTSD are supported by relatively less evidence than tier B treatments, many people do benefit from tier C treatments. New research findings are constantly being reported at conferences and in medical journals showing that some treatments currently supported by weak or inconclusive research findings in the medical journal literature may actually be more effective than previously believed.

The amount of time it takes to feel and function consistently better after starting any treatment or treatment combination, depends on many factors including how severe your PTSD symptoms are, whether you are dealing with more than one mental health problem or have a medical problem, the particular treatment of treatments you are using, the amount of stress you are under, your general state of health and how closely you've been following your plan.

Most medications and supplements take time to work so it may take several weeks to experience consistent improvement after starting a medication or a natural supplement. Information on how much time it usually takes for particular treatments to work is included in the treatment summaries.

Deciding when to change your treatment plan

The following questions will help you decide when to change your treatment plan.

How do I know if my current treatment plan is working?

If your symptoms of PTSD not severe most of the time your current treatment plan is probably working well. On the other hand, if your PTSD symptoms have not improved since starting a new treatment, your treatment plan clearly isn't working, or you may not be using a particular treatment in the most effective way. Some people take longer than others to respond to the same dose of a particular medication, natural supplement or the level of commitment to a mindfulness practice, a mind-body approach, or energy work. If your current treatment plan is helping to reduce your PTSD symptoms and function better at work, school and in your social life but you continue to struggle with PTSD, you may benefit from adjusting dosages (of a medication or natural supplement) or increasing the frequency of a mind-body practice, energy work, or another approach you've been trying, while continuing to follow the same general treatment plan as before. It is important to make decisions about changing or stopping your treatment plan on the basis of an accurate assessment of your PTSD symptoms. For this reason I encourage you to answer the questions in the same self-assessment inventory you used when deciding on your initial treatment plan. The results will help you to find out whether your PTSD symptoms are the same, worse or better than before.

Taking inventory of your symptoms will give you the information you need to decide whether to continue your current treatment plan, try something new, or stop treatment all together. Keeping a record of your answers will provide useful information about changes in your symptoms over time and which treatments are more effective.

If I'm not getting better how much longer should I wait before considering starting a new treatment?

The answer to this question depends on many factors that are different for each person. The amount of time needed to achieve consistent improvement in your PTSD symptoms in response to a particular treatment is listed under that treatment. In general, if a treatment you are currently using worked in the past it will probably be effective this time. Unless you have severe PTSD that is impairing your ability to work, study or be in a relationship, or you are experiencing serious side effects to a medication or natural supplement, I encourage you to continue your current treatment plan for several more weeks before trying something new.

How concerned should I be about side effects and what can I do if I get them? Making decisions about changing your treatment plan based on side effects has to do with how serious they are and how much they interfere with your ability to function. If you have a few mild side effects caused by a medication or a natural supplement that don't impair your ability to work, go to school, or interfere with other aspects of your life, your body may *get used* to these side effects fairly soon. On the other hand, if you are having side effects that interfere with your ability to function (e.g. sexual side effects, weight gain, problems with memory or concentration), it is prudent to stop your current treatment plan and try something new.

Depending on the medication or natural supplement that is causing side effects, changing the dosage or adding another medication or supplement can sometimes reduce or completely eliminate the problem. Of course, adding another medication or natural supplement can also cause new side effects. Before making any changes in your treatment plan aimed at reducing side effects, I encourage you to get expert advice from your psychiatrist or your family doctor.

When should I try something new in addition to my current treatment? How do I decide what to try?

As a general rule it is best to keep your treatment plan as simple as possible and avoid any combinations of treatments that cause potentially serious safety problems. If you are feeling and functioning better on your current treatment plan and your PTSD symptoms aren't severe, I encourage you to wait a little longer before trying something new. On the other hand, if you aren't feeling and functioning consistently better on your current treatment plan, or you are experiencing severe symptoms of PTSD, I encourage you to consider trying something new that may enhance the beneficial effects of your current treatment. Deciding whether to add a new treatment to your current treatment plan depends on the *likelihood that the change will result in improvement that would otherwise not take place.* Deciding whether to add another treatment to your current treatment plan also depends on whether the potential risk of side effects outweighs the potential benefits of starting a new treatment.

Before deciding whether to use two or more treatments at the same time I encourage you to first review the information in the treatment summaries to learn about combinations known to be effective and safe. In order to minimize the risk of side effects and potentially unsafe interactions please exercise caution when adding any new treatment to an existing treatment—whether it is a medication, a natural supplement or something else.

When should I stop what I'm taking and try something new or take no treatment at all?

If you are taking a quality brand natural product or a medication at the recommended dosage, or using a whole body, mind-body or energy therapy on a regular basis but you are not feeling and functioning consistently better, it may be time to discontinue your current treatment plan and wait before starting any new treatment. For example, and you are taking a medication or a natural supplement under the advice of a psychiatrist or an alternative medical practitioner, I encourage you to see your health care provider for advice on how to safely discontinue the medication (or supplement) before starting any new treatment. For the most part, gradually decreasing the dosage of a medication or supplement reduces the risk of side effects that can take place when abruptly stopping a treatment. In some cases, especially for less severe symptoms of PTSD, you may feel better after stopping a medication or a natural supplement.

By maintaining a healthy life style including regular exercise, getting enough sleep, following a stress management program, and maintaining a healthy diet, moderately severe symptoms of PTSD may improve even in the absence of treatment. However, if you are impaired by severe symptoms of PTSD, it is prudent to consider adding another treatment to boost the effectiveness of your current treatment plan, or to consider switching to an entirely new treatment.

Before doing either of these, I encourage you to first consult with a psychiatrist or experienced alternative practitioner for expert advice and guidance. When deciding whether to try any new treatment for PTSD use the same steps you followed when developing your initial treatment plan.

When should I see a psychiatrist or alternative healthcare practitioner for expert advice including questions about dosages, concerns about adverse effects, or to find out whether I have a medical problem?

It is prudent to consult with a psychiatrist or an experienced alternative healthcare provider if you are experiencing side effects caused by a medication or a natural supplement. I strongly encourage you to see your family physician or other medically trained healthcare provider if you think you have a medical problem in order to get a thorough evaluation and to find out whether your medical problem is making your PTSD symptoms worse or interfering with your response to treatment.

Repeating the steps until you find a treatment plan that *works for you*

Sometimes it is necessary to try many different approaches in order to get to a treatment plan that works. Every time you go through the process of deciding on a treatment plan you will have a better understanding of your PTSD symptoms and how they change over time. You will also have useful insights about treatments that work as well as ones that *don't work*.

When evaluating your PTSD symptoms, you can use the same self-assessment questionnaire as many times as you need to. By saving your answers you can track how your PTSD symptoms respond to changes in your treatment plan. This information will help you decide whether to continue on your current treatment plan, try something new or stop treatment all together.

If you have not experienced consistent reduction in the severity of your PTSD symptoms after trying two different treatment plans, I encourage you to seek advice from a psychiatrist or other mental health care provider with experience treating PTSD. *Finally—and I can't emphasize this point strongly enough—if you experiencing severe symptoms of PTSD, if you have another serious mental health problem, I encourage you to seek immediate medical care.*

Summary of main points

Below I summarize the most important points in this book including key steps involved in developing a safe, effective and affordable treatment plan based on your history, symptoms, preferences and circumstances:

- **If you are experiencing severe symptoms of PTSD or you are thinking about harming or killing yourself, or if you have another serious mental health problem that is impairing your ability to function, I urge you to *seek urgent medical care at the nearest hospital or emergency room*.**

- This book is offered as a practical resource on the safe and effective alternative treatments of PTSD.

- Alternative medicine sometimes called 'complementary and alternative medicine or CAM—consists of approaches that are currently not used in mainstream Western medicine (also called 'biomedicine' and 'allopathic medicine').

- Integrative medicine is a person-centered approach to care that incorporates mainstream Western medical treatments and CAM approaches.

- Integrative mental health care is the area of integrative medicine aimed at optimizing emotional and mental wellness and treating specific mental health problems.

- If you've recently been hospitalized or evaluated in an emergency room for severe symptoms of PTSD and you are functioning better now, this book will help you find reliable information about alternative treatment approaches.

- If you *have* a medical problem that has not been diagnosed, is not being treated, or has recently been getting worse, I encourage you to see a physician or other medically trained healthcare professional before making *any* changes in your current treatment plan or starting any new treatment. Medical problems that often occur together with PTSD include cardiovascular disease, arthritis, hypertension and autoimmune disorders.

- The first step in developing a treatment plan that is right for you involves taking inventory of your PTSD symptoms using the self-assessment questionnaires provided on the companion website. Your answers will help you better understand the nature and severity of your PTSD.

- After taking inventory of your PTSD symptoms, the next step is to carefully review the evidence for various treatments and to identify those treatments that make sense for you.

- The next step involves deciding whether to start treatment on your own or to work with a healthcare provider.

- Moderately severe symptoms of PTSD sometimes respond to changes in life style such as stress management, better sleep and exercise.

- Severe PTSD symptoms seldom respond to life style changes alone, and may require long-term treatment with a medication, a natural supplement or a medication and natural supplement in combination. Decisions about combining two or more medications or supplements should be based on scientific evidence and safety considerations. *If you are experiencing severe PTSD symptoms, I strongly encourage you work closely with a psychiatrist or psychotherapist who can evaluate you and advise you on a treatment plan that is appropriate for you.*

- Even if you need a medication or a natural supplement in order to feel and function better, making positive lifestyle changes such as exercising more often, adequate sleep, and a stress reduction program, can help you function better.

- Recall that none of the currently available alternative treatments for PTSD are supported by the highest level of evidence (i.e., tier A). Thus, when developing your treatment plan first consider using tier B modalities. If you have already tried several tier B treatment approaches without benefit, I encourage you to review the detailed information in this book on those treatments you've tried to make sure you previously used a quality brand (i.e. if it is a natural supplement) at the recommended dosage and for the recommended period of time. If you've already tried a mindfulness, mind-body or energy approach, but were disappointed in the results, I encourage you to review the information on that particular approach to make sure you used it in a way and for a period of time that would be expected to yield beneficial results.

- If you discover that you did not try a tier B treatment at the optimal dosage and duration, I encourage you to try that treatment again. This time making sure you use the recommended dosage of a quality brand for the recommended amount of time. If you previously tried a mindfulness, mind-body or energetic approach that is known to be beneficial for PTSD, but without success, I encourage you try that approach again, this time closely following recommendations on frequency and duration of treatment that would most likely achieve beneficial results.

- An important consideration is deciding whether to try one treatment or a combination or two or more treatments at the same time. *Examples of beneficial combinations as well as unsafe combinations to be avoided* are included in the detailed descriptions of the various treatments.

- If your PTSD symptoms are not responding consistently to your initial treatment plan *after following it for the recommended amount of time,* I encourage you to find a psychiatrist or other medical trained provider to obtain diagnostic tests in order to make sure that a medical problem is not exacerbating your symptoms or interfering your response to treatment.

- If your PTSD symptoms do not improve after you've followed your treatment plan for a period of time after which you should expect beneficial results, I encourage you to consider switching to a different treatment, preferably one that also belongs to tier B. The amount of time in which you should expect improvement in response to a particular treatment is discussed under each treatment. Depending on the severity of your symptoms, it may be helpful to continue your current treatment while adding one or more new approaches.

- Make sure you know about safety concerns associated with any treatment or treatment combinations you are considering. Safety problems are described under the specific treatments. *Before combining two or more treatments first review the comments on safe and effective treatment combinations as well as warnings pertaining to particular treatment combinations. It is always best to avoid combining two or more treatments that can potentially result in a toxic interaction.* If you decide to combine two or more treatments after reviewing the information in this book, I encourage you to first consult with a psychiatrist or other health care provider who is experienced in the treatment of PTSD for expert advice and guidance.

- It is important to take a close look at your PTSD symptoms from time to time—*even when your treatment plan is working well.* Doing a self-inventory by answering standardized questions will help you understand your PTSD symptoms better and determine whether you are experiencing significant new symptoms of PTSD or another mental health problem.

- Continue to modify your treatment plan on an on-going basis using an appropriate self-assessment inventory to document any changes in symptoms. Changes in your PTSD symptoms over time may call for changes in your treatment plan. If you are not feeling and functioning consistently better after trying at least two different treatments for the recommended period of time please seek expert advice from a psychiatrist or other mental health professional for formal evaluation and expert advice.

- If you are experiencing moderately severe symptoms of PTSD after trying at least two separate treatments, you may be able to remain at your current level of functioning after discontinuing treatment. Many people who experience moderate symptoms of PTSD benefit from life-style changes including regular exercise, improved sleep and stress management.

Going deeper

After reading this e-book on alternative treatments of PTSD you may want to learn more. You can find in-depth information in my other books:

- *An Integrative Paradigm for Mental Health Care: Ideas and Methods Shaping the Future*, **Springer, 2019**

- *Textbook of Integrative Mental Health Care*, **Thieme Medical, 2006**

- *Integrative Mental Health Care: A Therapist's Handbook*, **Norton 2009**

- *Complementary and Alternative Treatments in Mental Health Care*, **American Psychiatric Association, Inc. 2006**

- *Chinese Medical Psychiatry: A Textbook and Clinical Manual*, **Blue Poppy Press, 2000**

You can find links to all of my books, as well as many full-text articles and conference presentations on my website http://progressivepsychiatry.com/

Finding quality products and services on the Internet

After you've decided on the treatment plan that makes sense for you the next step is to find quality products and services that you can use. This section includes valuable internet resources that will help you select safe, effective and affordable products and services. Some of the resources listed are free while others charge a subscription fee.

General resources on complementary and alternative treatment approaches

- **Progressive Psychiatry** http://progressivepsychiatry.com/ This is the author's website. It includes a comprehensive list of on-line resources on both mainstream mental health care and complementary and alternative medicine (CAM) approaches. You can find several full-text articles published by Dr. Lake as well as presentations made at various conferences over the years. The site also includes a blog on integrative mental health care and links to all of Dr. Lake's books.

- **The National Center for Complementary and Integrative Health (NCCIH)** https://nccih.nih.gov is part of the National Institutes of Health (NIH). NCCIH is dedicated to exploring complementary and alternative healing practices in the context of rigorous science, training complementary and alternative medicine (CAM) researchers, and disseminating authoritative information to the public and professionals. The site contains extensive reviews of research on all non-medication treatment approaches. A citation index contains over 200,000 citations of studies on all areas of non-conventional medicine indexed in the National Library of Medicine beginning in 1966. The section includes valuable advice on how to find qualified practitioners of alternative and integrative medicine. The site includes information **en Español.**

Resources on dietary supplements (no fee)

- **National Institutes of Health Office of Dietary Supplements** https://ods.od.nih.gov/ provides an extensive on-line library of dietary supplement fact sheets for widely used herbals and other natural products. Different versions are available for consumers and health professionals. The site includes frequently asked questions (FAQs) and links to scientific monographs. The site includes some information **en Español.**

- **Medline Plus Supplement Information** https://medlineplus.gov/druginformation.html is a service of the U.S. National Library of Medicine, National Institutes of Health. It includes a comprehensive library of on-line monographs on prescription drugs as well as herbals and other natural product supplements. Each monograph includes safety information on adverse effects and interactions. The site also includes free mental health screening tools, educational brochures, videos and podcasts on common mental health problems.

- **Drugs.com** https://www.drugs.com/ includes a comprehensive library of on-line monographs on prescription medications and natural products including extensive information on adverse effects. It includes an on-line tool for checking interactions. Different versions are available for consumers and health professionals. The information on the site is also available **en Español**.

- **National Herbalists Association of Australia** https://www.nhaa.org.au Founded in 1920, the National Herbalists Association of Australia is the oldest natural therapies association in Australia, and the only national professional body of medical herbalists. Their mission is to serve and support membership (Medical Herbalists and Naturopaths) and to promote and protect the profession and practice of herbal medicine. This website is a portal to on-line resources covering all aspects of herbal medicine as well as complementary and alternative medicine in general. It includes links to valuable resources on research, nutrition, herbals and other natural product supplements, professional associations, educational resources, and reputable distributors and suppliers of herbals and other natural products.

- **The World Health Organization's (WHO) traditional medicine portal** https://www.who.int/traditional-complementary-integrative-medicine/en/ provides a traditional medicine fact sheet and links to worldwide health care resources. WHO seeks to promote international collaboration and cooperation in the study and use of traditional healing approaches in mental health care.

Resources on natural products and other non-medication treatments (fee)

- **ConsumerLab.com**   https://www.consumerlab.com/

  provides independent test results and information to help

  consumers and healthcare professionals evaluate health,

  wellness, and nutrition products. ConsumerLab is a

  certification company and enables companies of all sizes to

  have their products voluntarily tested for potential

  inclusion in its list of Approved Quality products and bear

  its seal of approval. The site is a valuable consumer

  resource for evaluating different natural products and

  brands and identifying brands that are both safe and

  effective.

- **Natural   Medicines**

  https://naturalmedicines.therapeuticresearch.com   is   a

  subscription service that provides valuable information on

  natural products and other non-medication approaches.

  Like Consumerlab.com, Natural Medicines provides

  independent reviews of supplements that are authoritative

and easy to read. The site provides links to valuable databases on natural products and other approaches. It also includes consumer monographs, patient handouts and offers continuing education credit on different topics to health professionals.

- **Herb Research Foundation** http://www.herbs.org/hrfinfo.html includes expert compilations on specific herbals that contain carefully selected articles, studies, and discussions by experts that are available as downloads or in print form. The work of the Herb Research Foundation is based on its dedicated holdings of more than 300,000 scientific articles on thousands of herbs.